# Understanding Acid-Base Disorders

This tutorial was developed while I was a medical student at the University of California, San Diego. Acid-Base disorders are common clinical problems encountered in both the outpatient and inpatient setting. Understanding the pathophysiology as well the clinical management for patients is not only fun and rewarding, but ensures proper patient management.

# Introduction (pg 5-7)

## Background

## Buffers
- HCO3- Buffer System
- Non-Bicarbonate Buffers
  - Intra Cellular Buffers
  - Hgb Buffer
  - Bone

# The Kidney's Role in Acid Base Homeostasis (pg 8-10)

## Reabsorption

## Replenishment
- Titratable acidity
- NH4+ Excretion

# Compensatory Responses (pg11-15)

## Background
- Metabolic Acidosis
- Metabolic Alkalosis
- Respiratory Acidosis
- Respiratory Alkalosis
- Davenport Diagrams

# Etiologies (pg 15-31)

## Metabolic Acidosis
- Hyperchloremic Metabolic Acidosis
  - GI causes
  - Renal Failure
  - Renal Tubular Acidosis
  - Distal (type 1) Renal Tubular Acidosis
  - Proximal (type 2) Renal Tubular Acidosis
  - Type 4 Renal Tubular Acidosis
  - Urine Anion Gap
- Anion Gap
  - Metabolic Causes
  - Ketoacidosis
  - Exogenous causes
  - Delta Delta (Δ/Δ) and Poisoning and the Osmolar Gap

## Metabolic Alkalosis
- Background
  - Volume Depletion
  - Aldosterone Excess
  - Hypokalemia
- Etiologies of Metabolic Alkalosis
  - Loss of GI fluids
  - COPDers
  - Diuretic Use
  - Volume resistant metabolic alkalosis
  - Urine Chloride Test

## Respiratory Acidosis
- Non-Pulmonary Causes
- Pulmonary causes
  - Acute
  - Chronic

## Respiratory Alkalosis
- Pulmonary Causes
- Non-Pulmonary Causes

# Step by Step Approach to Assessing Acid Base Status (pg 31-38)

# Sample Cases (pg 39-44)

# References (pg 45)

# Introduction

**Background Info:**

Let us begin by developing a comfortable background in acid base chemistry and physiology

pH will be the most important parameter when working on acid base vignettes

pH is a measure of [H+] and is defined as the negative logarithm of [H+]=-log[H+]

There are 2 factors that determine the [H+] and they are pCO2 and [HCO3-]

These 2 values are the important parameters to measure when assessing a patient's acid base status

CO2 as we all know is the breakdown product of glucose and it accumulates in our blood until we exhale it via our lungs

We Measure the [CO2] as the partial pressure of CO2 in plasma; pCO2

This CO2 is in equilibrium with HCO3- and can be described by the following equation:

$$CO_2 + H_2O \longleftrightarrow HCO_3^- + H^+$$

HCO3- in this equation acts as a buffer and hence controls the amount of H+ that is in flux from various sources to manage immediate changes in pH

Ionic buffers in solution tend to be weak acids that will take on extra H+ to minimize the drastic effects of pH changes that would occur outside their presence

Since the immediate effects of an offset of pH are managed by HCO3- we see that there can be a major drop in its concentration

If the disturbance is from the left side and it's from CO2 then it must be a respiratory disorder

If the disturbance is from the right side of the equation and either due to HCO3- or H+ then it must be metabolic

Important to distinguish between a processes (-osis); alkalosis/acidosis and states of the blood (-emia); academia and alkalemia

**Buffers:**

5 main buffer systems in our body

Plasma: HCO3-, phosphate, Hemoglobin, and plasma proteins

Non-Plasma: Bone

### HCO3- Buffer System:

The most important buffer system in the body

Can be regarded as a weak acid conjugate base system where HCO3- is the conjugate base that can take H+ to form CO2 and H2O

$$CO_2 + H_2O \longleftrightarrow HCO_3^- + H^+$$

The uncatalyzed reaction kinetics are normally very slow

With the use of the enzyme *Carbonic Anhydrase* the rate is amped up drastically

The reaction will follow the basic rules of Le Chatelier's Principle where an increase on the left will lead to an increase on the right and a decrease in any of the products on the right will lead to a decrease on the left

## Non-Bicarbonate Buffers:

- 80% of the non-$HCO_3^-$ buffering capacity is due to HgB and its actions are mediated by the amino acid Histidine side chain
- Albumin is the most important of the plasma proteins and again uses Histidine as its active side chain
- Phosphate $(PO_4)^{3-}$ is the last and least important of these…its actions are just like $HCO_3^-$ and are governed by basic weak acid conjugate base chemistry but the concentration in the plasma is so low that it is note effective on an absolute scale

## Intra Cellular Buffers:

- These buffers are important in maintaining the pH within cells
- They are mostly inorganic phosphates and proteins who mediate their actions via histidine side chains and phosphates
- Hemoglobin is also an intracellular buffer but will be discussed separately because it is the only intracellular buffer that has a significant impact on plasma pH

## Hgb Buffer:

- $HCO_3^-$ diffuses into the RBC where it attaches to Hgb
- In the lungs where $PO_2$ is high $O_2$ combines with Hgb and releases the $HCO_3^-$ which is reduced to $CO_2$ and exhaled
- Approximately 20% of the buffering capacity of blood is handled by the Hgb system

## Bone:

- Bone represents a site of non-plasma buffering
- Bone buffering is not important in the acute phase but is important in the chronic phase
- Performs its buffering action via the release of $CaCO_3$
- In the setting of kidney failure this can lead to osteodystrophy

## Review Question:

Which of the following statements is the most correct?

a- pH is a measure of [H+] and is defined as the logarithm of [H+]
b- The 3 determinants of acid base status in the $HCO_3^-$ buffer system are $PCO_2$, [$HCO_3^-$], and [H+]
c- The concentration of $CO_2$ in our bodies is controlled mainly by metabolism
d- Via the action of $CaCO_3$ bone also contributes to the buffering reaction in the acute setting

Answer: B, we know that from the $HCO_3^-$ buffer equation that the 3 determinants of acid base status are $PCO_2$, $HCO_3^-$, and H+. Regarding the incorrect answers we know that pH=Negative logarithm of [H+], that $CO_2$ is a byproduct of metabolism but it concentration is maintained by the buffer system and ultimately via exhalation through the lungs. Lastly bone is an important buffering site but it is only involved in the chronic management of acid base status.

**Review question:**

Which of the following statements most correctly describes the buffer systems in our bodies

a- The phosphate buffer is the most important non-HCO3- buffer in our plasma because of its simple non-protein based chemistry
b- The HCO3- buffer is the most robust and important buffer system in our plasma and is catalyzed by the enzyme carbonic anhydrase
c- Intracellular buffering is mediated primarily by hemoglobin
d- Tyrosine is the amino acid side chain that governs acid base status in protein buffers

**Answer:B**, The HCO3- buffer system is the most important buffer system in our body and will be the one that you concentrate on when you solve problems later on. The phosphate buffer does act like the HCO3- buffer but is very low in concentration in the plasma, intracellular buffering is performed by many proteins which can include Hgb but that is not the primary one except in RBCs, and lastly Histidine is the side chain that primarily regulates acid base reactions for proteins

**Review question:**

Using the CO2 equilibrium question predict what will happen to the concentration of H+ and HCO3- when there is an increase in the PCO2 from 40mmHg to 55mmHg such as in the case of hypoventilation

a- Decreased HCO3- and increased H+
b- Decreased HCO3- and decreased H+
c- Increased HCO3- and increased H+
d- Increased HCO3- and decreased H+

**Answer:C**; We know that according to Le Chatelliere's principle that an increase of PCO2 will lead to an increase in both HCO3- and H+

# The Kidney's Role in Acid Base Homeostasis:

The function of the kidney wrt HCO3- management is two-fold: **Reabsorption and Replenishment**:

**Reabsorption:**

When plasma is filtered by the kidney HCO3- builds up in the tubular lumen

Via the enzyme *Carbonic Anhydrase* the reclaimed HCO3- is reduced to CO2 which passes freely into the proximal tubule cells

Via the action of intracellular *Carbonic Anhydrase* it is HCO3- is regenerated

The basolateral side HCO3-/Na transporter pumps HCO3- into the peritubular capillaries

Note that there is also an H+ that is generated in this process which is pumped back into the lumen

The important transporters are the **Na+/H+** exchanger in the proximal tubule and the **H+ATPase** in the distal nephron

These transporters details may appear to be small font but will become important when understanding Renal Tubular Acidosis

Important to realize that this process is not simply reclaiming the filtered HCO3- but is converting it to CO2 initially and then regenerating a HCO3- molecule which is pumped back in to the plasma

The majority of the HCO3- reabsorption occurs in the proximal tubule while the remaining is in the loop of Henle

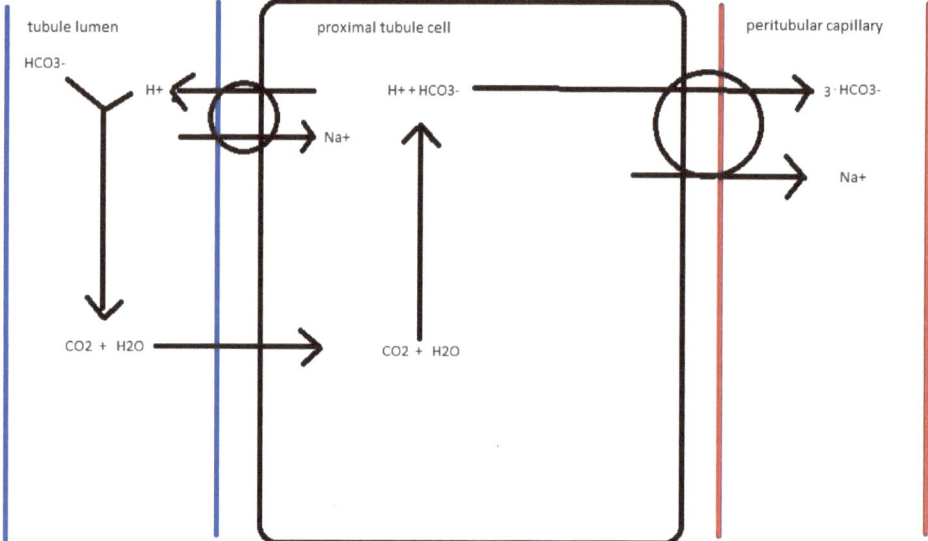

**Figure A**

### Replenishment:

In the setting of chronic acidosis where there is constant depletion of $HCO_3^-$ stores the kidney steps in to manage this problem via 2 mechanisms; titratable acidity and ammonium generation

### Titratable acidity:

When the $HCO_3^-$ levels fall the role of phosphate buffers become more important $(HPO_4)^{2-}$ serves as a $H^+$ acceptor and allows the Carbonic Anhydrase mediated reaction to continue inside the proximal tubule cells and hence there is generation of $(H_2PO_4)^-$ ions in the collecting tubules

Other anions become important also and these include sulfate, chloride, and in the case of diabetics acetoacetate and hydroxybutyrate

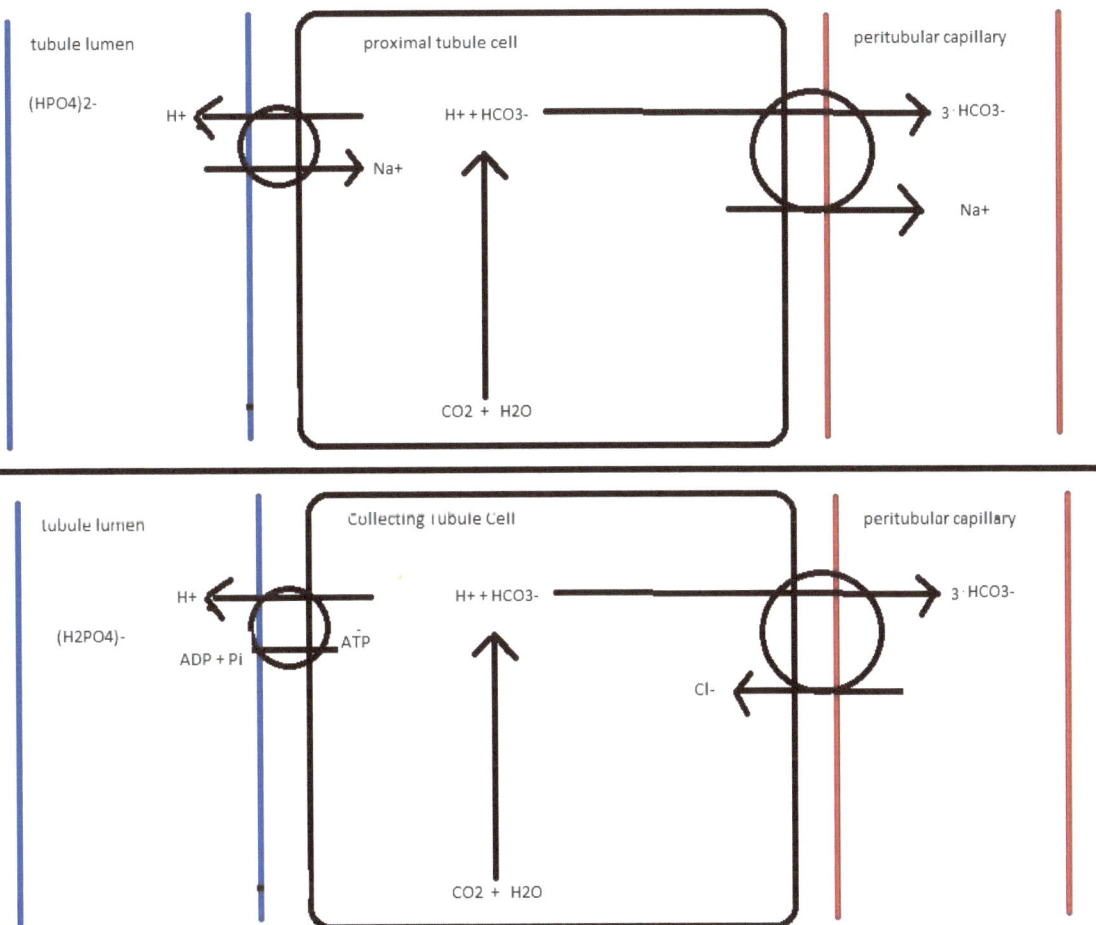

As the titratable acid $(HPO_4)^{2-}$ works its way down the tubular lumen the pH gradient increases drastically and ir is reduced to $(HPO_4)^-$

**Figure B**

## NH4+ Excretion:

The second important mechanism is NH4+ excretion

This mechanism has been debated for decades now but some of the more recent data show the following mechanism:

Glutamine serves as a metabolism precursor for the formation of HCO3- and NH4+

Glutamine is broken down in proximal tubule cells to HCO3- which is pumped into the peritubular capillaries and NH4+ which is pumped into the nephron tubule

Use Figure C below to better understand what is going on during this process

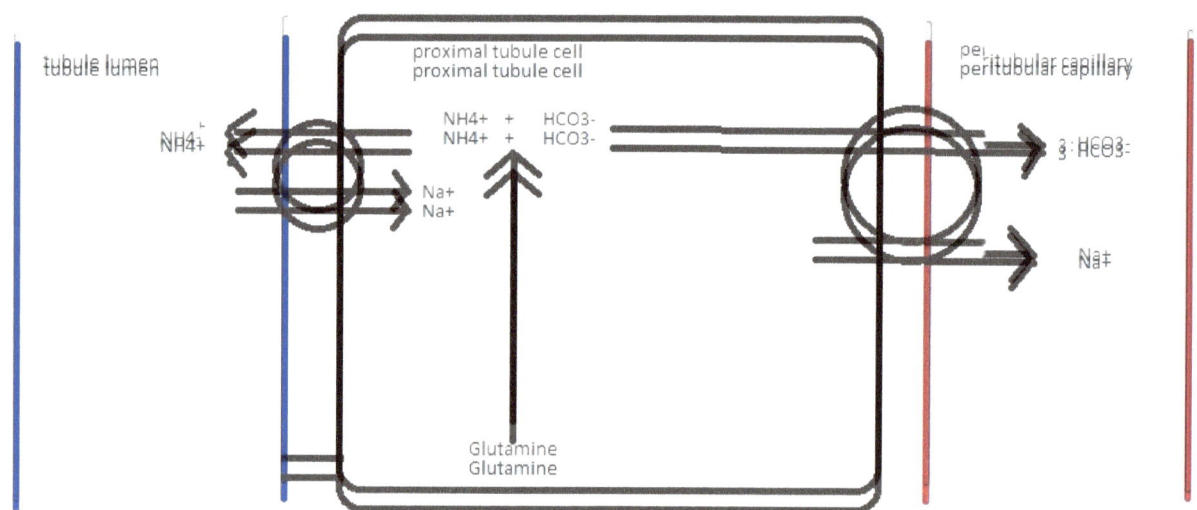

Figure C

## Review Question

Which of the following statements most correctly describes the management of HCO3- and H+ regulation by the kidney?

a- NH4+ excretion is one of the modes by which the kidney replenished HCO3- and is from the synthesis of Glutamine

b- Titratable acid represent a mode by which the kidney generates HCO3- when it is low in plasma and of the many ions that are used Phosphates are the most important

c- The mechanism of HCO3- reabsorption involves passive diffusion of the HCO3- ion across the proximal tubule wall and ATP mediated transport into the peritubular capillary

d- Na+H+ exchangers are what mediate the acidification of urine along the entire length of the nephron

Answer: B; ACD are incorrect because NH4+ excretion is the product of Glutamine breakdown not synthesis, the mechanism of HCO3- reabsorption does not involve passive diffusion of HCO3- but actually breakdown to CO2 and reformation to HCO3- via the enzyme Carbonic Anhydrase. Lastly, NaH+ exchangers are what are used in the proximal tubule and H+ATPase are used in the distal tubule.

# Compensatory Responses:

## Background:

A compensatory response is defined as a response that fights and attempts to minimize how a respiratory and/or metabolic insult affects the [H+]

It is important to distinguish compensatory responses from primary responses, which are usually the insults, and corrective responses which are what ultimately correct the pH on the long run

Let us look at some examples of primary insults and assess what the compensatory response will be

There are important quantitative ways to measure these changes though they will be discussed in the problem solving section at the end.

In this section we will focus on understanding the concepts and physiology of the 4 primary insults: metabolic and respiratory acidosis/alkalosis:

### Metabolic Acidosis:

We can use a generic example of a patient in the ICU who developed sepsis with an accumulation of lactic acid and a resulting metabolic acidosis with an increased [H+] load

When looking at the equilibrium buffer reaction in blood:

$$CO_2 + H_2O \leftrightarrow HCO_3^- + H^+$$

We see that the initial insult will push the equilibrium to the left and we will have a decrease in $HCO_3^-$ and for a moment an increase in $CO_2$...but since the chemoreceptors in the CNS respiratory center are very sensitive to these changes hyperventilation will kick in within minutes to decrease the $CO_2$ load and hence we will have a decrease in $pCO_2$ from normal

The final compensatory response is hyperventilatory induced hypocapnea

This process will come to an end when the initial insult is removed and the $HCO_3^-$ level has returned to normal.

In this case when the patient is treated properly in the ICU and there is a decreased load of H+ on the system

Please Refer to diagrams D and E to better understand where we are on the Davenport Acid Base Map

### Metabolic Alkalosis

We can use a generic example of excess vomiting in which a patient has been vomiting for the last several hours and has lost significant amounts of gastric contents and hence gastric acid (H+)

When looking at the equilibrium buffer reaction in blood:

$$CO_2 + H_2O \leftrightarrow HCO_3^- + H^+$$

We see that the initial insults involves a removal of H+ from the right side of the equation and hence the equilibrium is pushed to the right and we see an increase in $HCO_3^-$ levels.....but since the chemoreceptors in the CNS respiratory center are very sensitive to the changes in $HCO_3^-$ they decrease the respiratory rate to conserve $CO_2$ in the bloodstream

Hence the final compensatory response is a rise in $PCO_2$

This process will come to an end when the initial insult is removed and the HCO3- level has returned to normal.
In this case it is when the patient stops vomiting and the body resumes to conserve it's H+ and reduce its HCO3- generation
Please Refer to diagrams D and E to better understand where we are on the Davenport Acid Base Map

**Respiratory Acidosis**
Let us use the example of the patient with the opiate overdose who develops profound hypoventilation secondary to decreased respiratory drive and an accumulation of CO2 in the bloodstream
When looking at the equilibrium buffer reaction in blood:
CO2 + H2O ←→ HCO3- + H+
We see that equilibrium is shifted to the right and we develop an increase in [H+]
Since the respiratory center itself cannot be used to compensate for the increased acid load it is the kidney this time that does it in the chronic phase
This process will come to an end when the initial insult is removed. In this case the administration of Naloxone, and opiate antagonist will allow the respiratory rate to return to normal
Please Refer to diagrams D and E to better understand where we are on the Davenport Acid Base Map

**Respiratory Alkalosis**
Let us use the example of a mountain climber at altitude who is hyperventilating to maintain proper levels of PO2. He is also blowing off large amounts of CO2 and has hence developed low PCO2 levels
When looking at the equilibrium buffer reaction in blood:
CO2 + H2O ←→ HCO3- + H+
We see that the drop on the left pulls the equilibrium in that direction hence we see a drop in HCO3- levels and H+
To conserve HCO3- it will be kidney that is ultimately responsible for minimizing H+ excretion and increasing HCO3- loss…this can also be facilitated by the administration of acetazolamide, a Carbonic Anhydrase Inhibitor to catalyze this process
Please Refer to diagrams D and E to better understand where we are on the Davenport Acid Base Map

**Davenport Diagrams:**
There are several methods that can be used to either determine or memorize these compensatory responses.

One can always use the Davenport diagrams that were used throughout respiratory and renal physiology

When using the Davenport Diagram always start from the normal

You can use the **rule of 4's;** pH=7.4, HCO3-=24, PCO2=40

From there determine where you will be moving

If there is a primary metabolic disturbance then you will initially move along the metabolic line to a new PCO2 and then come to pH 7.4 via a respiratory compensation

If there is a primary respiratory disturbance you will move up or down the isobar initially and then come to pH7.4 via a renal compensation

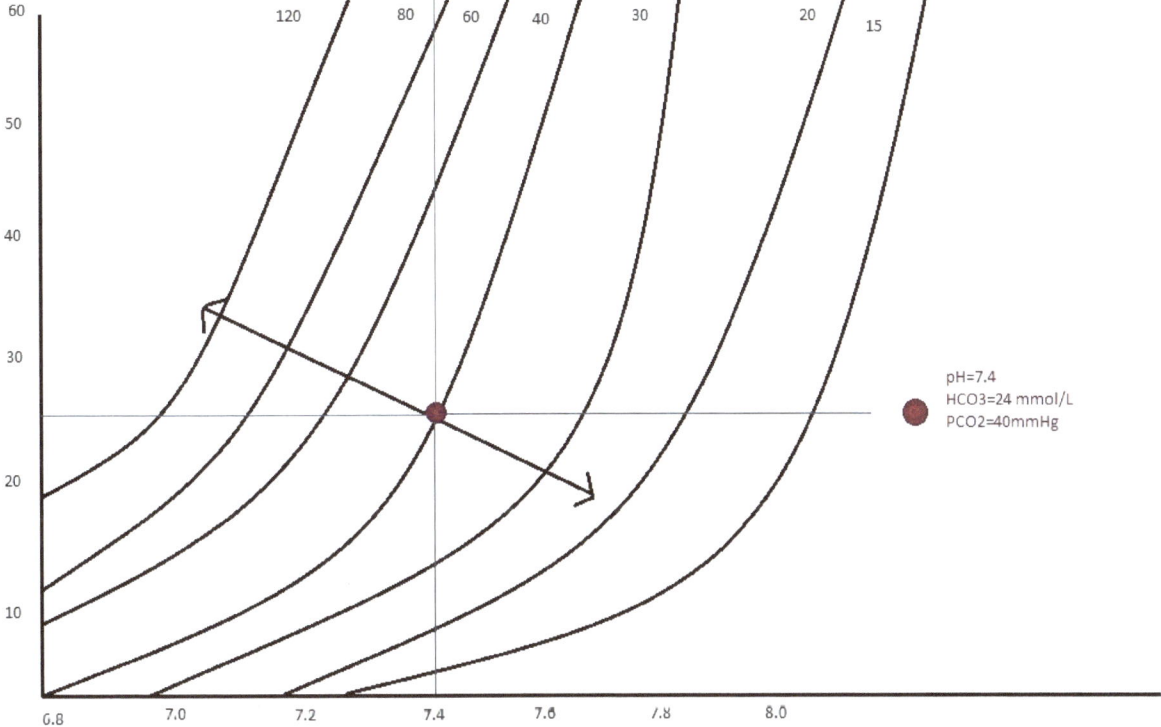

**Figure D**

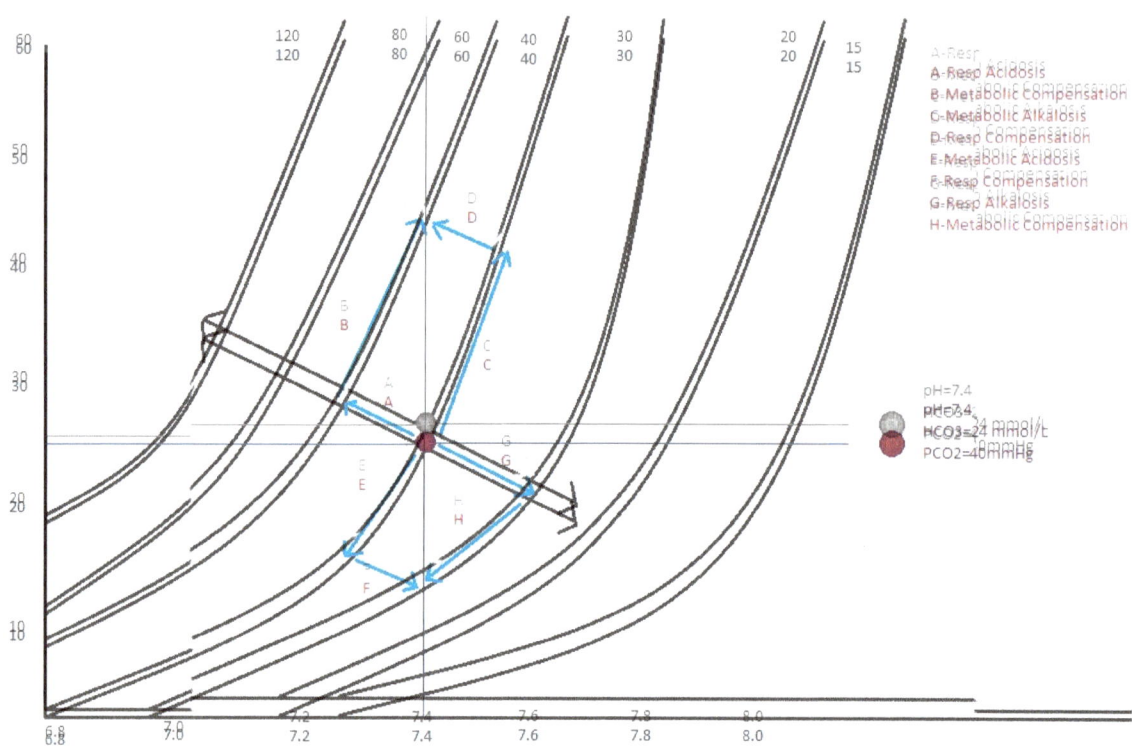

### Figure E

Students may also use this summary chart if they wish to memorize the compensatory changes

| Primary Disturbance | Compensatory Response |
|---|---|
| Metabolic Acidosis | Decreased PCO2 |
| Metabolic Alkalosis | Increased PCO2 |
| Respiratory Acidosis | Increased HCO3- |
| Respiratory Alkalosis | Decreased HCO3- |

### Review Question:

Using the davenport diagram which of the following values seems like a reasonable position for a person who overdosed on morphine in the acute phase ?

| PCO2 | HCO3- | pH |
|---|---|---|
| a-60mmHg | 28 | 7.25 |
| b-60mmHg | 22 | 7.35 |
| c-30mmHg | 22 | 7.55 |
| d-30mmHg | 28 | 7.55 |

**Answer**: A; from the example we have determined that this patient has opiate induced hypoventilation. Thinking about the pathophysiology for a few moments we realize that hypoventilation will lead to increased CO2 retention and hence a buildup of H+ and HCO3- in the acute setting. Using the Davenport diagram we move along the metabolic line in the direction of acidosis where we see that PCO2=60mmHg and HCO3-=28 is a reasonable answer

## Review Question:

A person who has just moved to a high altitude town has been hyperventilating for several days now. Which of the following set of values most likely represents his acid base status?

| PCO2 | HCO3- | pH |
|---|---|---|
| a=60mmHg | 28 | 7.40 |
| b=60mmHg | 23 | 7.23 |
| c=30mmHg | 22 | 7.40 |
| d=30mmHg | 28 | 7.55 |

Answer: C, when we think about the question we realize that this person has altitude induced hyperventilation. We know that this response decreases his PCO2 levels as he breathes this off and he is in respiratory alkalosis. Given the fact that he has been at altitude for a few days we know that this has given his kidneys some time to decrease the HCO3- load in his body and help bring his pH back to normal. The point that corresponds the best to this is C where we have a normal pH, a decreased HCO3- level and a low PCO2 level.

# Etiologies

There will be 4 major categories of acid base etiologies discussed here
They will be metabolic acidosis, metabolic alkalosis, respiratory acidosis, and respiratory alkalosis

## Metabolic Acidosis

Metabolic acidosis is defined as acidemia with low HCO3- and low PCO2 (Thomson et al)
Acidosis will be described from a hypobicarbonatemic view so all definitions and mechanisms will assessed from the viewpoint of decreased HCO3- levels
Acidosis can be caused by excessive input of H+, decreased excretion of H+, or loss of HCO3-
Remember to use this equation if you get confused: $CO_2 + H_2O \leftrightarrows HCO_3^- + H^+$
There are numerous ways to organize the numerous etiologies of metabolic acidosis though the most convenient one I find is the division into Hyperchloremic Metabolic Acidosis (AKA normal anion gap) and Anion Gap Metabolic Acidosis

### Hyperchloremic Metabolic Acidosis:

Hyperchloremic metabolic acidosis derives its name from the mechanisms that cause a hyperchloremic state that is since there is a drop in $HCO_3^-$ levels there must a subsequent elevation in $Cl^-$ ions to maintain electroneutrality

There are 3 main causes of hyperchloremic metabolic acidosis and they are diarrhea, renal tubular acidosis and renal failure

Looking at figure F below we can see that there are instances where we have a metabolic acidosis that leads to a decrease in $HCO_3^-$ levels and an increase in $Cl^-$ levels

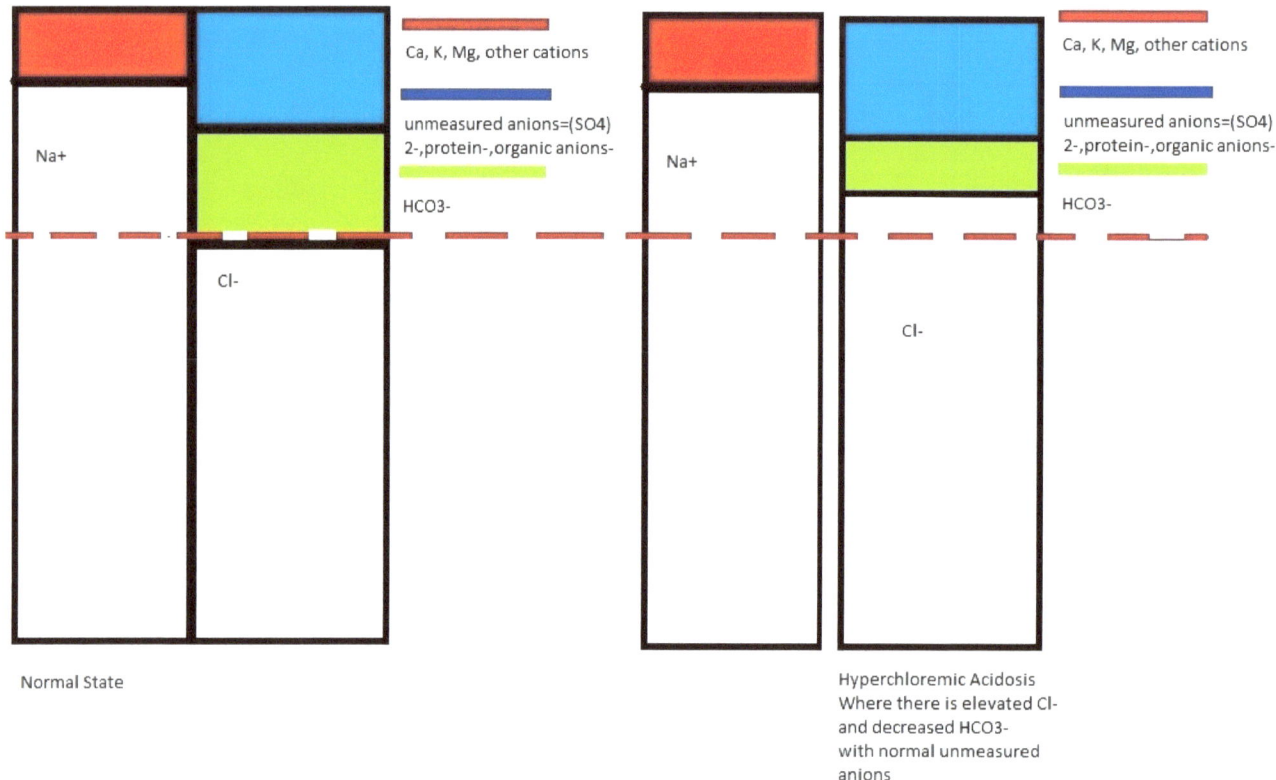

**Figure F**

**GI causes:**
From basic GI physiology we know that there are many modes through which $HCO_3^-$ leaves the body and in return $H^+$ is returned to the bloodstream

Diarrhea is the most common cause of gastrointestinal acidosis

Mechanism involves increased $HCO_3^-$ loss through the GI lumen, increased $H^+$ reabsorption into vasculature as a result of $HCO_3^-$ loss, and ECF contraction from water loss leading to RAAS activation and subsequent hypokalemia/acidosis.

Look at Figure G to better understand where the ions are traveling

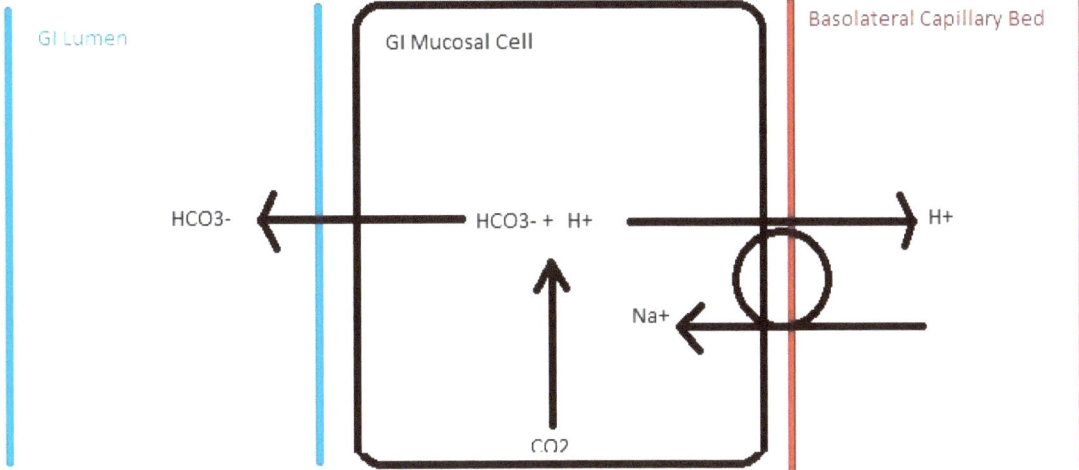

**Figure G**

**Renal Failure:**
Renal failure will lead to not only decreased HCO3- filtration but also decreased ammoniagenesis
Mechanisms involves damage to both the glomerulus and the tubule
Glomerular damage leads to decreased GFR and hence decreased HCO3- reabsorption
Tubular damage leads to decreased ammoniagenesis
The net damage is a reduction in the total number of functioning nephrons

**Renal Tubular Acidosis**
Renal Tubular Acidoses are a group of disorders that lead to a failure of the kidney to acidify the urine and hence there is a buildup of H+ in the bloodstream and a resultant Acidosis
There are 3 subtypes: 1,2,4

**Distal (type 1) Renal Tubular Acidosis**
Can be caused by familial, autoimmune, drug induced, nephrogenic, or idiopathic causes
The distal kidney loses its ability to generate the large H+ gradients and reabsorb the HCO3- that it needs
This leads to a decrease in the amount of titratable acidity and ammoniagenesis
Hypokalemia is always present
Overall a very rare cause of RTA

**Proximal (type 2) Renal Tubular Acidosis**
Caused by proximal tubule dysfunction that leads to HCO3- wasting from decreased reabsorption

- Causes are varied and include amyloidosis, multiple myeloma, cystinosis, Wilson's disease, etc.
- Hypokalemia is always present
- Much more common children than in adults

### Type 4 Renal Tubular Acidosis:
- Caused by either decreased aldosterone secretion, decreased sensitivity to aldosterone, or administration of aldosterone antagonists such as spironolactone
- Hyperkalemia will be present and is necessary in the diagnosis (useful to distinguish from types 1&2)
- Mechanism of acidosis is complicated but one theory suggests that hyperkalemia which directly leads to suppression of $NH_4^+$ production (Abelow et al)
- Most common RTA in adults usually in diabetics and patients with adrenal disease such as Addison's or AIDS induced adrenal disease

### Urine Anion Gap
- An useful calculation that one can do to determine if the cause of a hyperchloremic non elevated anion gap acidosis is either from diarrhea or renal tubular acidosis is the urine anion gap calculation.
- The premise of this calculation is the $NH_4^+$ levels will be the unaccounted cations and they will force the calculation to be either positive or negative
- UAG=Na + K-Cl
- (+)UAG=RTA
- (-)UAG=Diarrhea

### Review Question:
With regard to GI causes of acidosis which of the following is incorrect

a- the excess secretion of $HCO_3^-$ into the GI lumen and the subsequent pumping of H+ into the bloodstream leads to metabolic acidosis
b- ECF loss from diarrhea also leads to a RAAS induced hypokalemic/acidotic state from excess K+ losses
c- The pancreas is also a source of $HCO_3^-$ excretion under normal circumstances with an impetus from gastric expulsion of contents
d- Osmotic diarrhea is the most common cause

Answer: D, all are true except D because an osmotic diarrhea would only pull H2O out of the lumen and not affect the $HCO_3^-$

## Review Question:
All of the following are true of renal tubular acidosis except:
a- Type 1 RTA is the least common subtype and can present with hypokalemia
b- Type 4 RTA is the most common subtype in adults and can be distinguished from the other 2 by the presence of hyperkalemia
c- RTA is really an umbrella term that encompasses a large group of diseases that lead to acidosis
d- Type 2 RTA is the most concerning for children because the consequences of hyperkalemia are more pronounced in children

Answer: D; RTA type 2 is more common in children yet it causes a hypokalemia and not a hyperkalemia

## Anion Gap:
Anion gap is one of the most important topics to cover when assessing a patient with metabolic acidosis.

In blood serum there exist an equal number of anions and cations
As can be seen by this diagram below the relative amount of the 2 major anions Cl- and HCO3- is less than the major cation Na+.
The anion gap is conventionally calculated as Na-(Cl + HCO3)
This normal "anion gap" is usually between 8-16mEq/L
In the setting of an acidic insult on the system we see that the level of HCO3- can decrease and the level of "unmeasured anions" such as lactate ions can increase.
Hence when we use our anion gap equation Na and Cl will remain unchanged while HCO3 decreases leaving us with an elevated anion gap
When the anion gap is measured to be above 16mEq/L we need to start considering some high anion gap based metabolic acidosis etiologies
A simple mnemonic can be used to remember these etiologies: **MUDPILES**

Methanol
Uremia
DKA
Paraldehyde
Isoniazid (INH)
Lactic Acid
Ethanol
Salicylate

The three most common are DKA, lactic acidosis, and Renal Failure (Uremia)

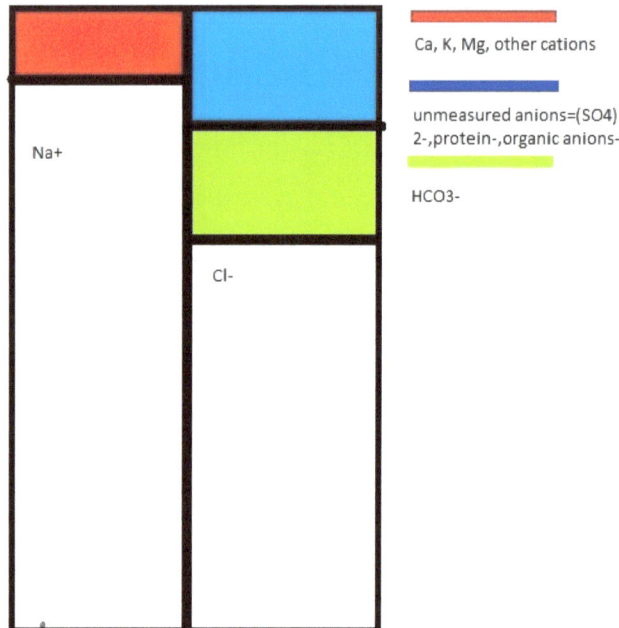

Normal relative concentrations of the major anions and cations in our blood

**Figure H**

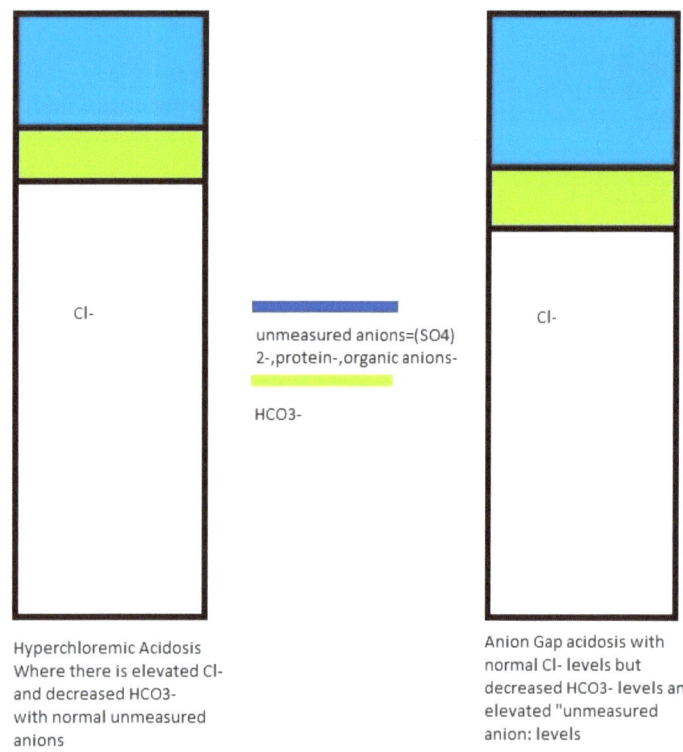

Changes in the anion band when there is a hyperchloremic vs. anion gap acidosis

**Figure I**

**Metabolic Causes:**
The 2 important ones to consider in this section are lactic acidosis and ketoacidosis
Lactic acidosis:
Lactate is the byproduct of anaerobic metabolism but is normally cleared by the kidney and liver
Lactic acidosis will develop when there is too much production of lactic acid.
If we think of the reasons why our bodies would switch to anaerobic mode they would include etiologies that lead to decreased organ perfusion such as sepsis, shock due to decreased cardiac output, seizures, prolonged exercise, alcoholism

**Ketoacidosis:**
This is particularly important in patients that are either type 1 diabetics or IDDM2 because they can enter into a state of diabetic ketoacidosis
Other causes include starvation and alcoholic ketoacidosis(which is really just vomit induced starvation from binge drinking)
Mechanism of acidosis involves the production of ketone bodies which contribute H+ to the plasma
Mechanisms also includes a contraction of the vasculature from the loss of these anions to the urine and the subsequent osmotic effect and diuresis
The 3 ketone bodies that we are concerned with acetone, beta-hydroxybutyrate, and acetoacetate

**Exogenous causes:**
The 3 most common substances to be concerned about in the setting of metabolic acidosis include methanol, ethylene glycol, and salicylate
Methanol and Ethylene Glycol are metabolized in the same manner that ethanol is and hence produce formic acid and oxalic acid respectively.
The mechanisms involves the addition of an acid load and hence a drop in HCO3- levels
There are also the toxic effects of these organic acids also that need to be concerned for
Salicylate toxicity is also a concern but it additionally causes a respiratory alkalosis due to the pronounced hyperventilation that it causes (this is called a mixed disorder)

**Review Question:**

Regarding the mechanism of exogenous compound induced metabolic acidosis which of the following statements is correct

a- Oxalic acid which is the breakdown product of methanol causes an acidosis via donation of a proton to solution

b- Salicylate poisoning will lead to a mixed metabolic state including a metabolic alkalosis and respiratory acidosis

c- Ethylene glycol a constituent of antifreeze is a common mode of suicide can cause a metabolic acidosis via contribution of H+ to solution

d- Salicylate poisoning's mechanism involves solely the contribution of H+ to solution

**Answer:** C; oxalic acid is the breakdown product of ethylene glycol, and salicylate poisoning causes both a metabolic acidosis and a respiratory alkalosis via hyperventilation

## Delta Delta (Δ/Δ):

A useful calculation in the determination of a mixed state in the setting of an elevated anion gap acidosis is the delta delta ratio

Delta/delta Δ/Δ = (anion gap)/Δ(HCO3-) = (anion gap – normal gap)/(normal HCO3 – expected HCO3)

The topic of delta delta can be a bit complicated but in short it can be described as follows:

In the setting of an isolated metabolic acidosis we expect there to be a lowered HCO3- level and the presence of a particular anion gap.

Thus if we calculate that ratio of the anion gap to change in HCO3- level we should expect to see different etiologies causing different ratios to come out

In a normal non anion gap metabolic acidosis we expect this ratio to be less than 0.4 because we have a small numerator and a large denominator

In a pure metabolic anion gap acidosis we expect a larger numerator than before and hence the ratio can rise to above 1.0 but will remain less than 2.0

If we had a mixed state in which there was a contribution of HCO3- to the solution and the denominator begins to shrink as the numerator has increased this can raise the ratio to above 2.0

If we take for example a case of patient with diabetic ketoacidosis with an AG of 20 who has experienced severe diarrhea he would have lost more HCO3- than expected from the isolated metabolic acidosis alone. Mathematically this would force the denominator to crash even further

When the ratio is said to be above 2.0 then a mixed state should be suspected

The following chart can help summarize the important facts

| Delta Delta Ratio | Interpretation |
|---|---|
| Less than 1.0 | Mixed Anion and Non-Anion Gap Acidosis |
| Between 1.0 and 2.0 | Pure Anion Gap Acidosis |

| | |
|---|---|
| Greater than 2.0 | Mixed Anion Gap Acidosis and Met Alkalosis |

## Poisoning and the Osmolar Gap:

While on the topic of Anion Gap Acidosis it is important to consider intoxication with methanol and ethylene glycol

A useful calculation that can be used to help determine if these substances are present in the blood is the osmolar gap calculation.

The Osmolar gap takes into account all the osmotically active substances that are accounted for in a normal blood sample (Na, BUN, glucose) and subtracts them from the true osmolarity calculation

Osmolar Gap = measured osmolarity - calculated osmolarity

Measured osmolarity = from instrumentation

Calculated osmolarity = 2[Na] + [glucose]/18 + [BUN]/2.8

This gap is normally 5-10 but can be increased to 16-greater than 20 in the presence of nonionic osmotically active particles such as ethylene glycol and methanol.

## Review Question

All of the following situations will most likely have an elevated anion gap acidosis except for:

a - A pt brought in for vomiting after drinking some homemade whiskey
b - A pt brought into the emergency department after ingesting an entire bottle of "my grandmothers arthritis/blood thinning medicine"
c - A pt that has had diarrhea for the last 2 days
d - A teenager that has been complaining of abdominal pain polyuria and polydipsia brought in for "appearing to be out of it" and hyperventilation
e - A pt in the ICU that has required pressors for severe hypotension with a known history of "large kidney stone"

**Answer:** C; All of the cases represent classis high anion gap metabolic acidosis except for C which would be a cause of hyperchloremic acidosis and not a MUDPILES anion gap metabolic acidosis

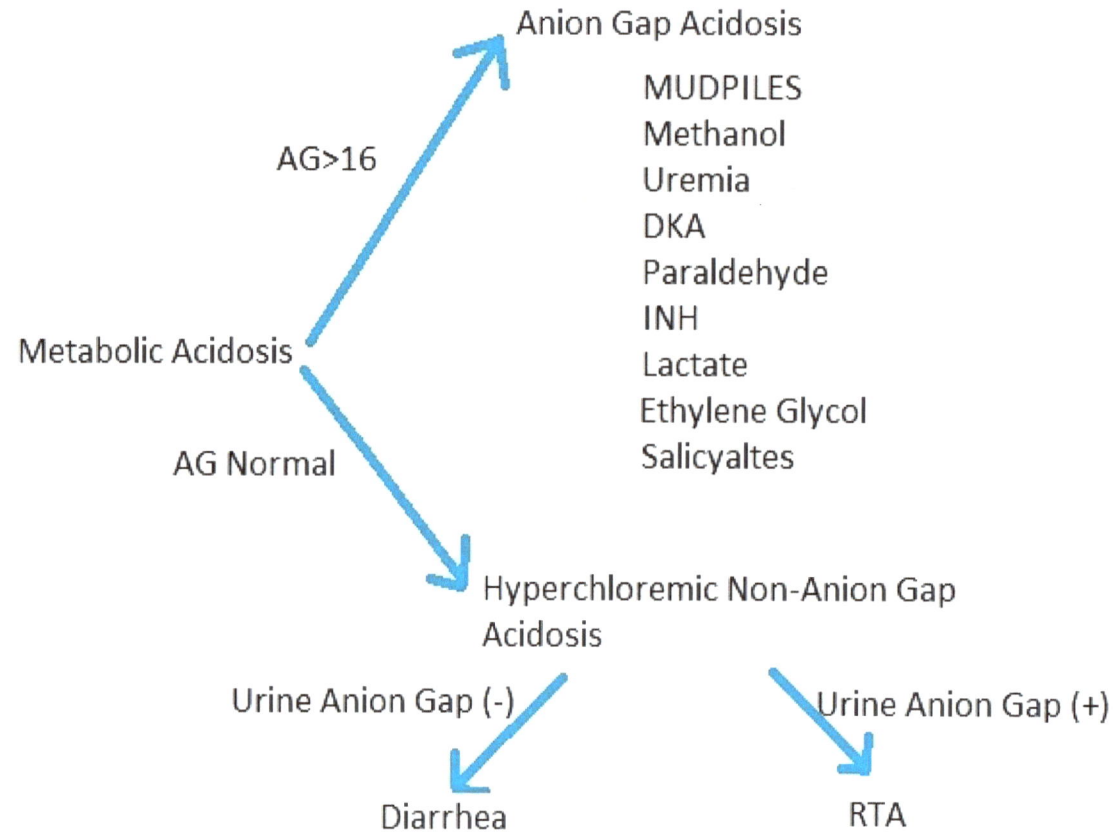

**Figure J**

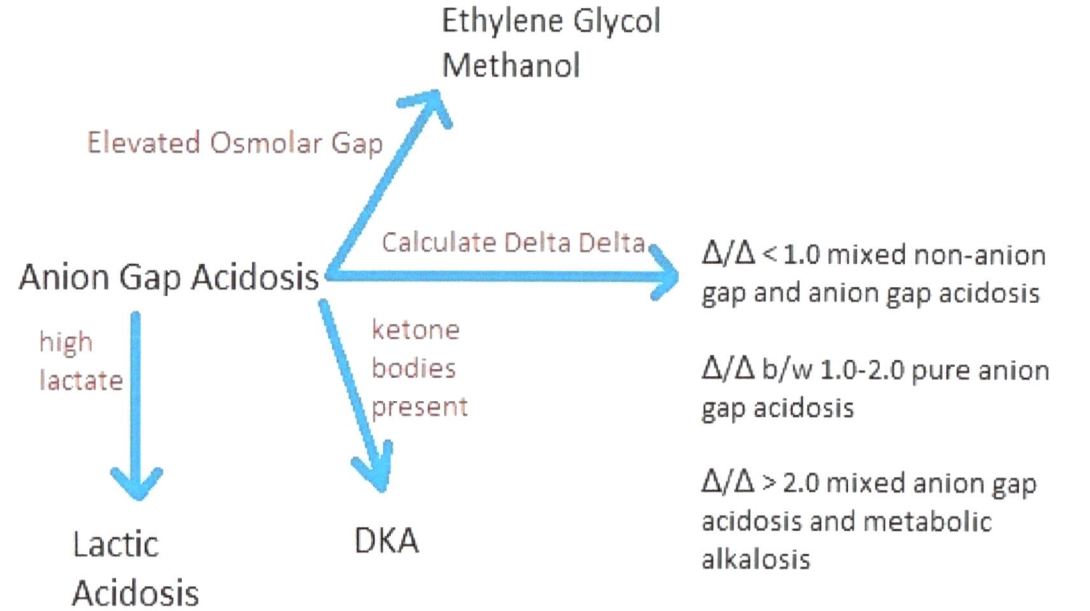

**Figure K**

## Metabolic Alkalosis

**Background:**

Metabolic Alkalosis is defined as an increase in HCO3- levels that lead to an alkalemia

There are 3 main causes that contribute to metabolic alkalosis and they are volume depletion, hypokalemia, and aldosterone excess

### Volume Depletion:

The mechanism of volume depletion induced metabolic alkalosis revolve around the effects of the RAAS system

Angiotensin II and sympathetic tone stimulates Na+/H+ exchange and Aldosterone exacerbates hypokalemia and hence alkalosis

Chloride concentrations in the tubular lumen have also been postulated to be a driving force in the reabsorption of HCO3-

### Aldosterone Excess:

Mechanism has been postulated to include increased H+ATPase activity in the collecting tubule

Mechanisms also involves the creation of a electrochemical gradient via the reabsorption of positively charged Na+ which leads to subsequent excretion of H+ into the lumen

This gradient also leads to the secretion of K+ into the lumen

### Hypokalemia:

The mechanisms involved in maintaining this increased threshold for HCO3- reabsorption include intracellular acidosis, increased H+K+ exchange, ammonium excretion, and reduced filtration rates

**Etiologies of Metabolic Alkalosis:**

There are 4 important etiologies to consider in the clinical setting: loss of GI fluids, mechanical ventilation in COPDers, volume resistant metabolic alkalosis, and diuretic therapy

### Loss of GI fluids:

2 common causes include vomiting and nasogastric suctioning of fluids

The stomachs response to decreased GI fluids is increased secretion of H+

Reviewing the mechanism of this generation we see that there is an equal amount of HCO3- pumped into plasma as there is H+ pumped into the stomach AKA the alkaline tide

### COPDers

In patients that have COPD respiratory acidosis is a common problem and as a chronic problem they tend to have elevated levels of HCO3-

When these patients need to be ventilated there can be a rapid drop in PCO2 back to normal without a subsequent drop in HCO3- levels and hence they qualify as metabolic alkalotics (remember that this an "artificial" alkalosis because there was no "process")

### Diuretic Use

Most common cause of metabolic alkalosis

Diuretics are commonly used to treat cirrhosis, heart failure, and nephrotic syndrome

Thiazides and loop diuretics are implicated

The mechanism can be understood if we understand the mechanism of diuretics

Diuretics cause a "saline flush" where the fluid that is diuresed from the body is saline rich but HCO3- poor

With the added effect of volume loss and HCO3- retention we understand how this state develops

### Volume resistant metabolic alkalosis

There are lots of conditions in which an intrinsic cause of increased aldosterone or mineralocorticoids with aldosterone receptor activity lead to hypokalemia and alkalosis

This is nothing more than a collection of diseases that lead to hypokalemia and a persistent alkalosis that are not responsive to fluids because hypovolemia is not at the root of the problem

The previous 3 etiologies mentioned are volume responsive

### Urine Chloride Test:

Urinary Chloride levels can be measured to help determine the etiologies

Urine Cl levels less than 15mmol/L signify a volume sensitive metabolic alkalosis

Urine Cl levels greater than 15mmol/L signify the very rare volume resistant metabolic alkalosis

Urine Na can be used place of Urine Cl though this can be misleading of the patient has just started using a diuretic

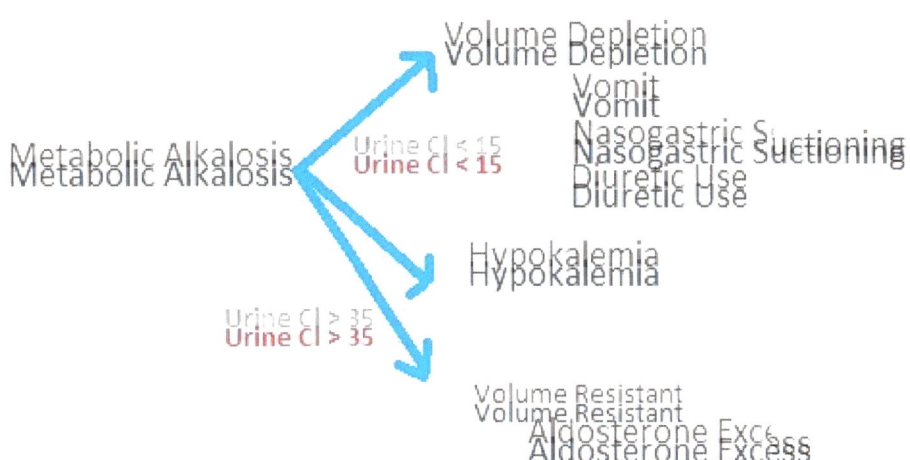

Figure L

## Review Question

Which of the following best correctly describes a mechanism of one of the metabolic alkalosis etiologies?

a- Conn's disease which is an aldosterone producing adenoma of the adrenal gland leads to volume resistant metabolic alkalosis via its secretion of excess amounts of aldosterone

b- COPDers on ventilators develop metabolic alkalosis as a result of volume contraction

c- CHF patients treated for exacerbations with diuretics are said to be volume resistant metabolic alkalotics because of the effects of aldosterone

d- Excess vomiting leads to a metabolic alkalosis via loss of HCO3- from gastric contents

Answer: A; B is wrong because COPDers on ventilators develop an alkalosis because they have an acute drop in CO2 without a drop in their elevated HCO3- levels, C is wrong because diuretic use , such as with loops and thiazides leads to loss of saline rich HCO3- poor water. D is incorrect because excess vomit leads to loss of H+ and a subsequent uncompensated for alkaline tide in the plasma

## Respiratory Acidosis

Respiratory acidosis is defined as a process that leads to an increase in PCO2 levels with a resultant acidosis

Important to remember that hyperventilation is a compensatory response to increased acid loads and it is hypoventilation that will lead to CO2 retention and acidosis

The 2 broad categories of respiratory acidosis etiologies are the pulmonary and non-pulmonary causes

### Non-Pulmonary Causes:

Drugs: opiates and benzodiazepines can lead to respiratory center depression

respiratory Center Trauma: strokes and tumors can damage the respiratory center and lead to respiratory depression

Spinal Cord Trauma: trauma to the spinal cord above C5 (remember C345 keeps the diaphragm alive) can lead to phrenic nerve dysfunction

respiratory Muscle Fatigue: Fatigue of the respiratory muscles secondary to overwork

**Pulmonary causes:**
There are once again 2 subdivisions and these are acute and chronic lung disease

**Acute:**
Acute disease includes pneumonia, asthma exacerbations, pulmonary emboli, and pulmonary edema

In healthy patients these acute causes usually result in hyperventilation and hypocapnea

In patients with chronic lung disease these acute exacerbations can lead to respiratory muscle failure and a resultant hypoventilatory induced hypercapnea and hence respiratory acidosis

**Chronic:**
Most common COPDers and of these much more likely to happen in patients with chronic bronchitis vs emphysema

These patients can remain hypercapnic for years

Part of this reason is that their respiratory muscles have fatigued and they cannot generate the resp drive necessary to exhale off the excess CO2

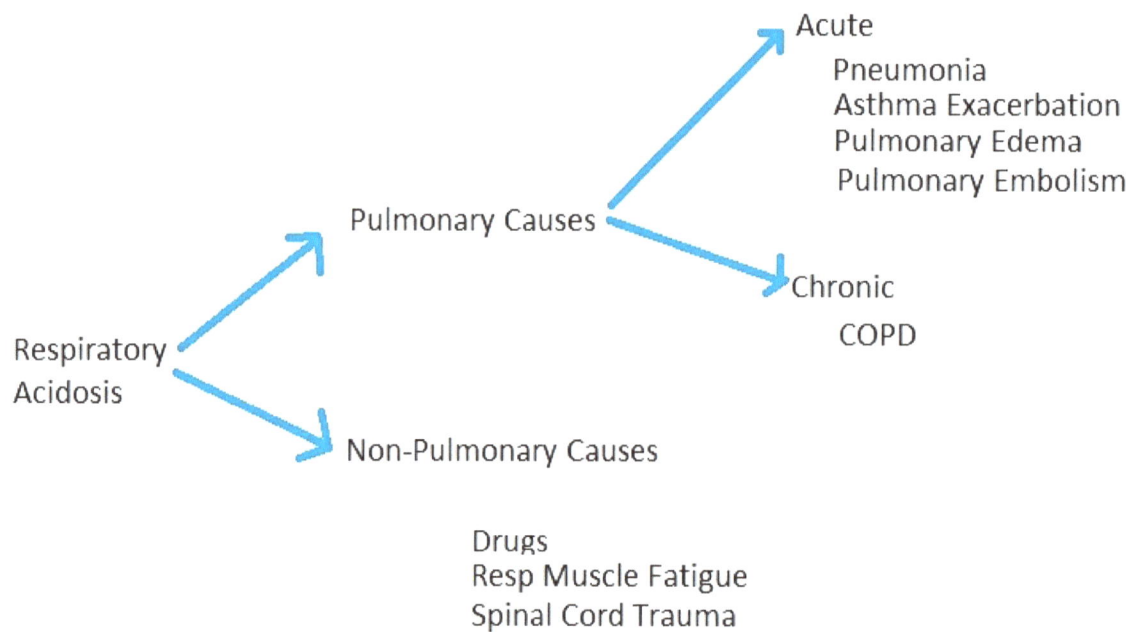

**Figure M**

**Review Question:**
*Which of the following is the most correct statement*
*a-asthma exacerbations in a young male patient will lead to hypocapnea because asthma is a chronic disease and these patients cannot mount the appropriate hyperventilatory response*
*b-CHF exacerbations that lead to pulmonary edema can be treated with diuretics and hence the only acid base concern for these patients is a contraction alkalosis*

*c-the patient will develop an initial hyperventilatory induced hypocapnea that will turn into a hypoventilatory hypercapnea if he has underlying lung disease and has resultant respiratory muscle fatigue*
*d-opiates and benzodiazepines are respiratory center stimulants and can lead to hyperventilation*
**Answer:** *C; A is wrong because even though asthma is a chronic disease it does not lead to resp muscle fatigue in a young patient and an exacerbation will lead to hyperventilation initially. B is partially corrects because diuresis will lead to a contraction alkalosis, but this is independent of the pulmonary edema. Lastly opiates and benzos are respiratory center suppressants and not stimulants*

## Respiratory Alkalosis

Let us briefly review the physiology and compensatory causes behind respiratory alkalosis
Hyperventilation leads to hypocapnea and an alkalosis
There are several causes that stimulate hyperventilation and they include arterial hypoxemia, pulmonary sense receptor stimulation, chemical/physical factors that directly affect the medullary center, and psychological factors
Hypoxemia severity directly correlates to ventilator response and is mediated by the central drive mechanism
Mechanoreceptors and irritant receptors also lead to an increase in respiratory drive and these are located in the alveolar walls
Direct stimulants to the respiratory center include salicylates, trauma, liver disease waste products, and trauma
Psychological factors including stress, fear, and pain can lead to hyperventilation
These are important factors to keep in mind as we begin to assess the clinical etiologies of respiratory alkalosis
The clinical etiologies can be lumped into 2 groups: pulmonary and non-pulmonary causes

**Pulmonary Causes:**
Recall the section in respiratory acidosis ; acute section where we listed some of the acute causes of respiratory acidosis.
These acute causes include pneumonia, pulmonary emboli, asthma exacerbation, pulmonary edema, and interstitial fibrosis
These all trigger hyperventilation and hence drive off the $CO_2$ from the blood leading to decreased $PCO_2$ levels
Remember from the last section that these conditions can progress to respiratory acidosis if there is underlying lung disease and the vent drive is blunted
It is crucial that patients with acute exacerbations superimposed on chronic disease be kept on high alert because it can lead to respiratory collapse and ultimately death

**Non-Pulmonary Causes:**

Etiologies include liver disease, sepsis, hemodialysis, brain lesions, salicylate toxicity, cyanotic heart disease, high altitude, pregnancy, psychological factors

The mechanisms are described briefly:

Liver disease: increased progesterone, estradiol, nitrogenous waste products and AV shunting

Sepsis: cytotoxic compounds released from the sepsis cascade

Hemodialysis: $CO_2$ diffusion from blood into the dialysis machine

Brain lesions: stroke, tumors and infection can lead to central hyperventilation

Salicylate toxicity: directly stimulates the medullary respiratory center

Cyanotic heart disease: hypoxemia secondary to right to left shunts

Altitude: hypoxia induced respiratory center escalation of respiratory rate

Pregnancy: progesterone stimulates the respiratory center

Psychological Factors: cerebral cortex mediated circuitry

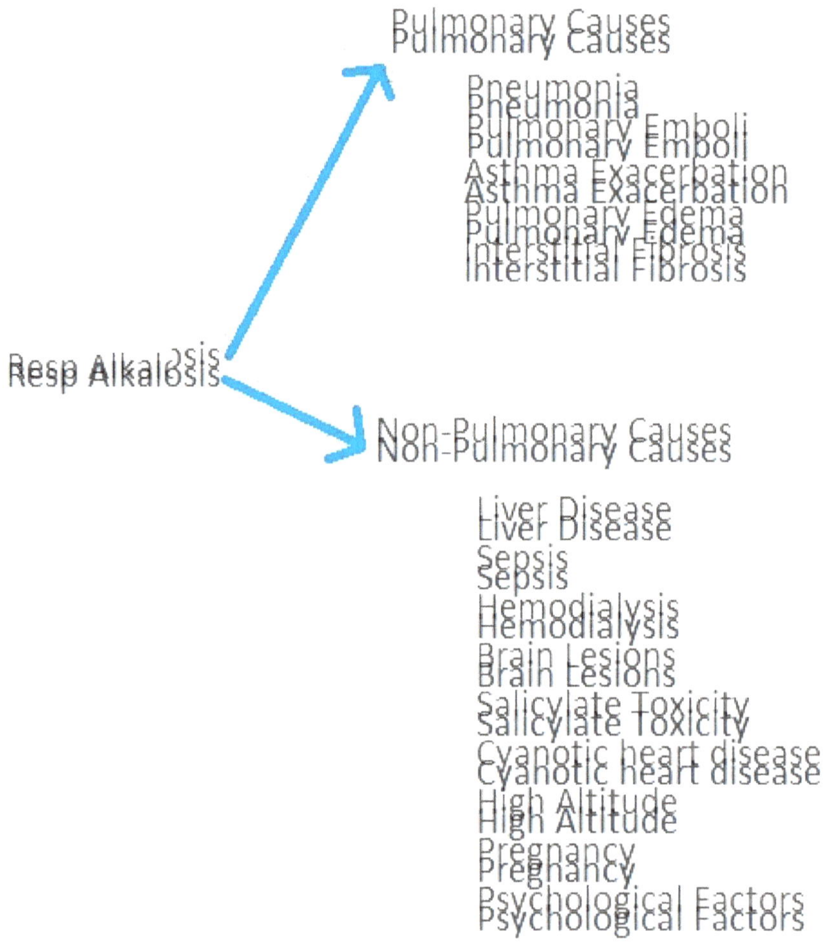

Resp Alkalosis
- Pulmonary Causes
  - Pneumonia
  - Pulmonary Emboli
  - Asthma Exacerbation
  - Pulmonary Edema
  - Interstitial Fibrosis
- Non-Pulmonary Causes
  - Liver Disease
  - Sepsis
  - Hemodialysis
  - Brain Lesions
  - Salicylate Toxicity
  - Cyanotic heart disease
  - High Altitude
  - Pregnancy
  - Psychological Factors

Figure N

## Review Question:

All of the following statements are true regarding respiratory alkalosis except:

a- liver disease and pregnancy induce a hyperventilatory response via progesterone
b- psychological factors though complicated to explain pathophysiologically are an important cause of hyperventilation
c- in the setting of sepsis hypoventilation is a common sign that can be observed with patients
d- a CNS insult such as a stroke can lead to either hyper or hypoventilation

answer: c; all are correct except for c, in the setting of sepsis the inflammatory mediators and cytokines will lead to respiratory center stimulation and hence hyperventilation

## Clinical Vignette Matching

Match the short clinical vignette with its appropriate simple acid base disorder

A- METABOLIC ACIDOSIS
B- METABOLIC ALKALOSIS
C- RESPIRATORY ACIDOSIS
D- RESPIRATORY ALKALOSIS

1- A 28 y/o pregnant female is brought to the ED for 2 day Hx of intractable vomiting
2- A 22 y/o male just started a mountain climbing trip has just passed 7,000 feet
3- 48 y/o male with terminal cancer brought in for excess opiate ingestion in an suicide attempt
4- 51 y/o male with IDDM2 brought to the emergency department for vomiting and hyperventilation

## Answers:

1- B; intractable vomiting will lead to a metabolic alkalosis
2- D; altitude induced hyperventilation will lead to respiratory alkalosis
3- C; opiate induced hypoventilation will lead to CO2 retention and hence respiratory acidosis
4- A; Diabetic Ketoacidosis is the result of unmanaged diabetes and is a cause of metabolic acidosis

# Step by Step Approach to assessing acid base status

**Step 1:** Clinical History: One of the most crucial steps in determining your differential diagnosis is the patient's history. Also important clues from the patient's physical exam including vitals should be incorporated into helping narrow down your differential diagnosis
**Step 2:** Determine from the pH if this is an acidemia or alkalemia
**Step 3:** Determine if the cause of the perturbation is metabolic, respiratory, or mixed

Use the following chart to determine in which direction your diagnosis will be headed

| Acidosis | pCO2 and HCO3- levels |
| --- | --- |
| Metabolic Acidosis | HCO3- < 24mmol/L |
| Respiratory Acidosis | pCO2 > 40mmHg |
| Mixed State | pCO2 > 40mmHg & HCO3- < 24mmol/L |
| **Alkalosis** | |
| Metabolic Alkalosis | HCO3- > 24mmol/L |
| Respiratory Alkalosis | pCO2 < 40mmHg |

| Mixed State | pCO2 < 40mmHg & HCO3- > 24mmol/L |

The diagram below will also help you visualize the following information

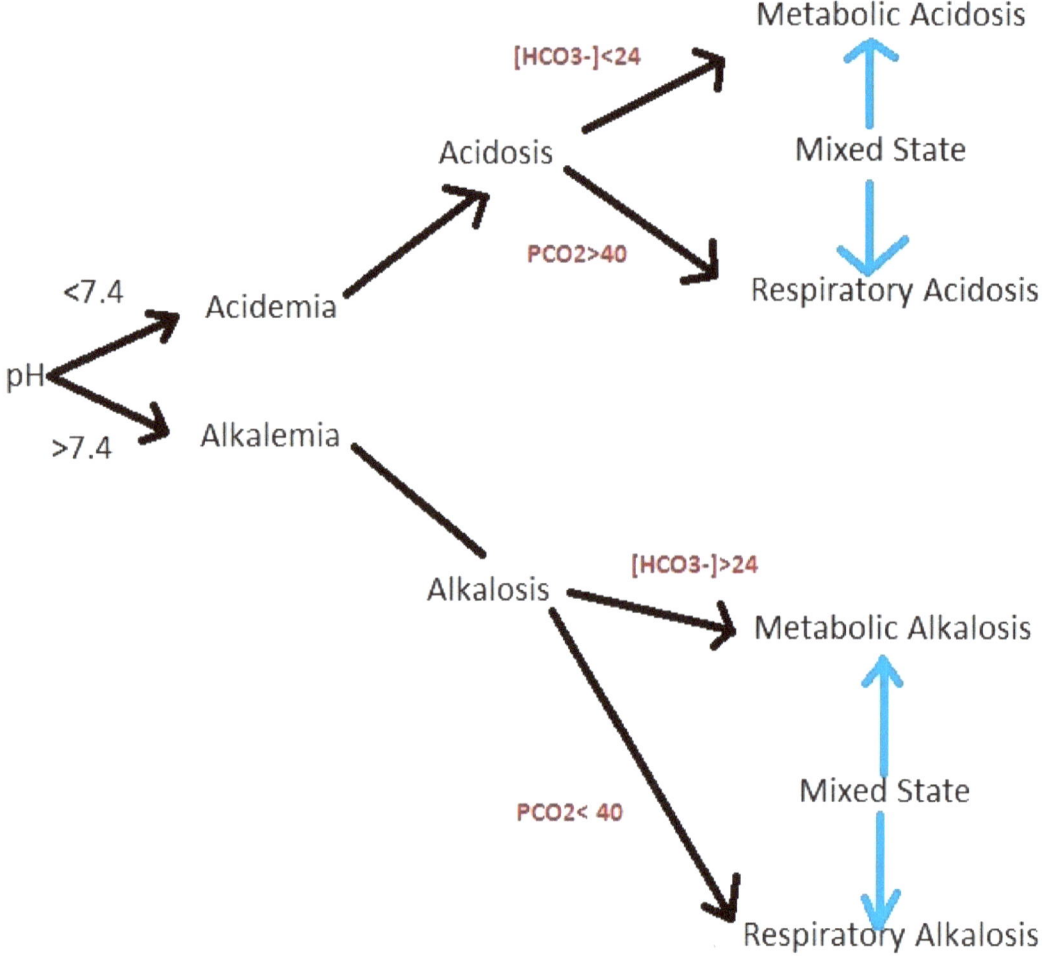

*Review Question:*

Which of the following sets of values represents a mixed respiratory and metabolic acidosis state?

| pH | PCO2 | HCO3- |
|---|---|---|
| a- 7.25 | 50mmHg | 24 mmol/L |
| b-7.25 | 50mmHg | 18 mmol/L |
| c-7.25 | 30mmHg | 18 mmol/L |
| d-7.50 | 30mmHg | 24 mmol/L |

**Answer:** B, This sample question is a bit like solving a problem backwards because it is asking you to predict what the lab values should be. First it is an academia so pH must be less than 7.40 that leaves us with choices a,b and c. Next we know that for a metabolic acidosis to exist the HCO3- levels have to be below 24mmol/L so that leaves us with choices b and c only. Last we know that if there is also a respiratory acidosis then there must be PCO2 value greater than 40mmHg and that leaves us with choice B.

**Step 4:** Determine if the level of compensation is appropriate to assess if there is a mixed state
The Following rules can be used to quickly determine if the level of compensation is appropriate. Remember you can also use the Davenport diagram as a map but do use the formulas for quick calculations.

| Primary Insult | Compensatory Change | Expected level of compensation |
|---|---|---|
| Resp Alkalosis | Drop in HCO3- | Acute: HCO3- decreases 2 per 10 fall in PCO2<br>Chronic: HCO3- decreases 5 for 10 rise in PCO2 |
| Resp Acidosis | Rise in HCO3- | Acute: HCO3- increases 1 per 10 rise in PCO2<br>Chronic: HCO3- increases 4 for 10 rise in PCO2 |
| Metabolic Acidosis | Drop in PCO2 | PCO2=1.5x[HCO3-]+ 8 +/-2 |
| Metabolic Alkalosis | Rise in PCO2 | PCO2 increases 0.5-1.0 per 1.0 rise of HCO3- |

(structure of this chart was borrowed from Benjamin Abelow's *Understanding Acid Base*)

*Review Question:*

The following ABGs are obtained for a patient that has had intractable diarrhea for 2 days
pH=7.20 HCO3=15 and PCO2=34mmHg. Is there an appropriate level of compensation?

**Answer:** we know from the vignette that this patient has a metabolic acidosis because they have a low pH and low HCO3-. We must now use the compensatory formula to determine if there is an appropriate level of compensation. Expected PCO2=1.5x(15)+8+/-2=22+8+/-2=28-32. Hence this patien'ts PCO2 is above the upper limit of normal and so there is not an appropriate level of respiratory compensation. We can think about this intuitively also without the use of numbers and think that with an original acid load insult we would expect the PCO2 levels to rise initially and quickly stimulate the resp center to amp up respiratory rate and "blow off" CO2. There is a mixed disturbance, i.e. an overlying respiratory acidosis that is competing with the metabolic acidosis.

*Important Caveats about compensation in the clinical setting though not likely to come up on exams because they will be testing major concepts and not subtleties:*

Before jumping to conclusions about there not being a proper compensatory response think about some of the following before you assume that there is a mixed state:

**Caveat 1: Timing**: the time frame of the clinical vignette and whether the respiratory or renal compensation has had enough time to become maximally effective

**Caveat 2: True under and overcompensators**: The approximation formulas used above statistically cover the majority of patients yet there are a few percent that will fall above and below these bounds

**Caveat 3: defects** in the compensatory pathways may be a true cause of an under or overcompensation

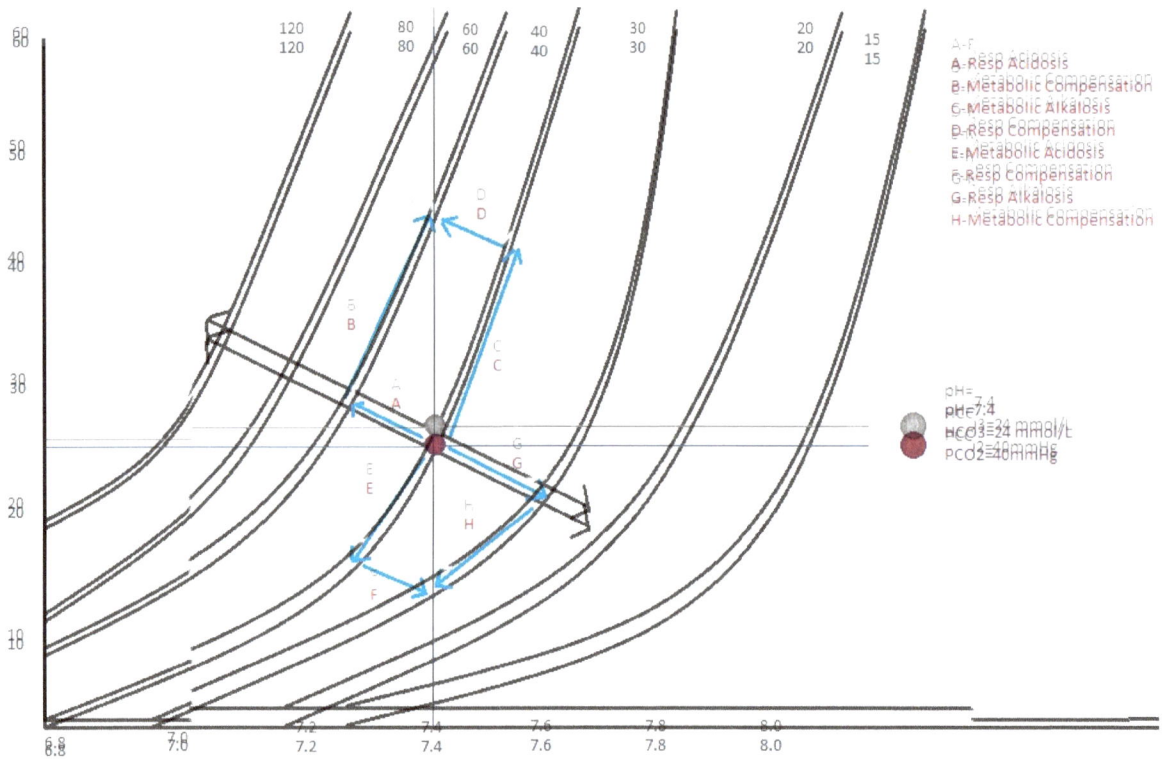

**Step 5:** Determine the most likely etiology of the disturbance. You can use the following diagrams to help guide your decision making process. It may be necessary to order additional tests to help narrow down the exact diagnosis. Often times you will already have a strong suspicion from the clinical vignette itself but you should always work through your logic and arguments carefully.

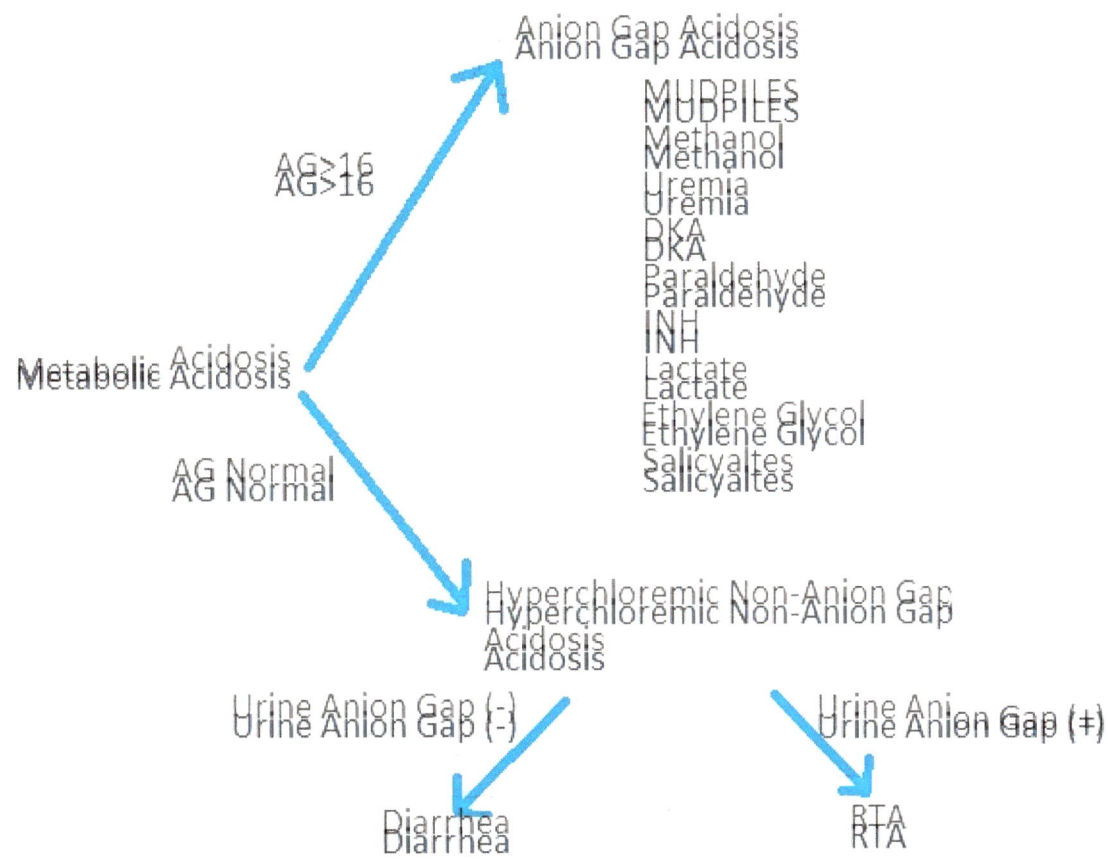

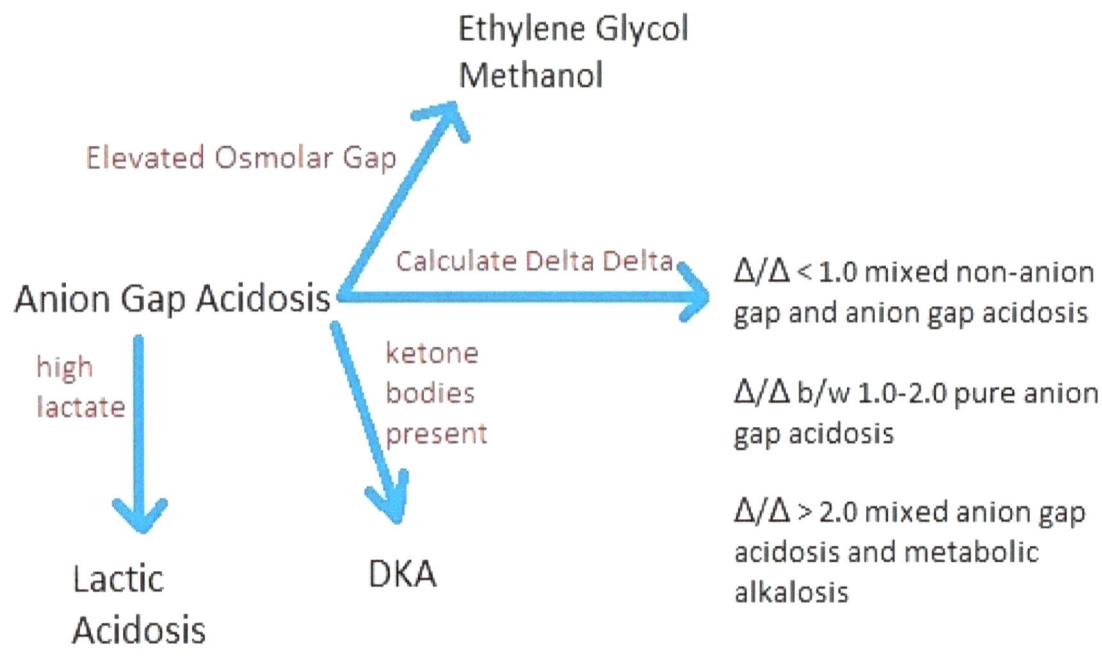

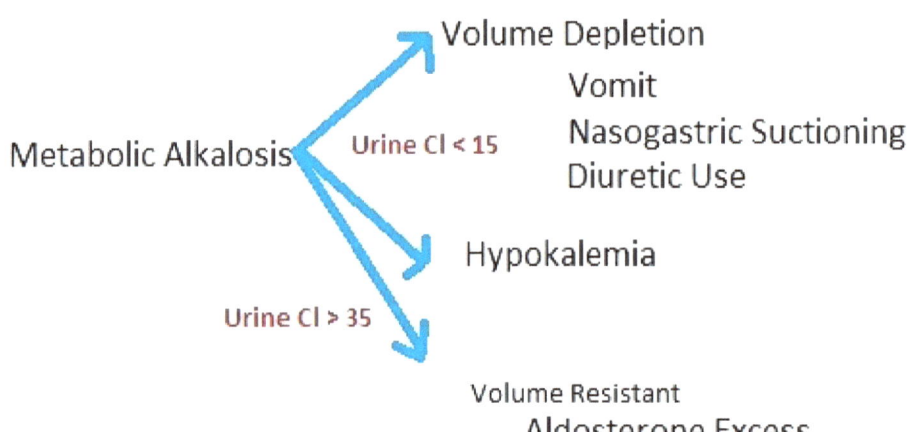

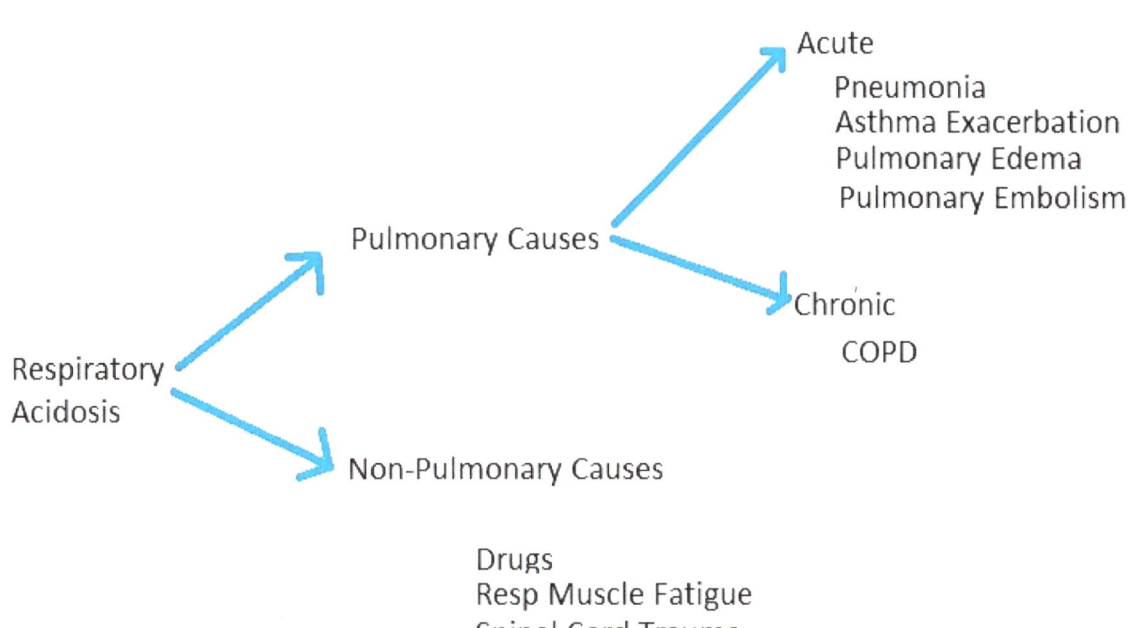

Resp Alkalosis

- Pulmonary Causes
  - Pneumonia
  - Pulmonary Emboli
  - Asthma Exacerbation
  - Pulmonary Edema
  - Interstitial Fibrosis

- Non-Pulmonary Causes
  - Liver Disease
  - Sepsis
  - Hemodialysis
  - Brain Lesions
  - Salicylate Toxicity
  - Cyanotic heart disease
  - High Altitude
  - Pregnancy
  - Psychological Factors

## Sample Problems:

The following are a series of sample problems that I have developed that you can work through to get a better feel for how to solve some of these acid base abnormalities. If the answer is clear right away then you don't need to work through the steps outlines above and if you have developed your own system of solving these problems then you do not have to confuse yourself any further. Also realize that in the clinical setting cases may not be so obvious and there may be several competing etiologies.

## Sample Case 1:

55 y/o female is brought into the emergency department following 8 hours of diarrhea in which she claims she has had 8 watery bowel movements. Laboratory values show pH=7.25, HCO3=18mmol/L, PCO2=34mmHg, Na=140, K=4.0, Cl=110. Vitals show HR=100, BP=100/70, temp=98.6, RR=22. What is her acid base abnormality? What is the etiology of her acid base disturbance?

**Step 1:** From the H&P we see that most important pieces of information are that she has had several watery bowel movements for the last 8 hours. This is concerning for HCO3- loss through the GI lumen.

**Step 2:** pH=7.25 therefore it is an acidemia

**Step 3:** Using the chart above we see that her HCO3- is low so she must have a metabolic acidosis. Let us now check to see if she has the appropriate level of compensation.

**Step 4:** Determine if there is an appropriate level of compensation: Since this is a metabolic acidosis we can use Winter's formula to determine this level of compensation: PCO2=1.5xHCO3 +8 +/- 2=(1.5x18)+8=35+/-2=33-37. Hence this patient has the appropriate level of compensation.

**Step 5:** Determine the etiology: Putting all this information together we have a patient who has had intractable diarrhea for more than a day. Her low HCO3- shows that she has a metabolic acidosis. Her resp rate and resultant hypocapnea are the compensatory response to exhale off the excess CO2. She has a normal anion gap of 12 and hence her metabolic acidosis is most likely either a GI cause or a renal cause. Given her History there is no reason to suspect a renal cause. By putting all the information together we can conclude that her primary insults was the diarrhea that lead to HCO3- loss and the development of the metabolic acidosis.

**Sample Case 2:**
A 43 y/o male with a known history of depression was found by his brother on the floor of his garage. He appeared confused, had slurred speech and appear to have vomited before being found. Labs were drawn in the emergency room: pH=7.28, PCO2=32mmHg, HCO3=18mmol/L Chemistry panel: Na140, K3.50,Cl 100 vitals Temp=99.2, HR=105, BP=110/85, RR=23. What is the etiology of his acid base disturbance?

**Step 1**: From the H&P we can conclude that this patient probably ingested some substance and may be intoxicated. There is also a set of abnormal lab values

**Step 2:** pH=7.28 therefore this is an acidemia. We must now determine if it is resp or metabolic

**Step 3:** Using the chart provided above we determine that there is a metabolic acidosis due to the fact that there is a low HCO3- . Let us now assess what the compensatory response should be and whether it is sufficient.

**Step 4:** Determine if there is an appropriate level of compensation. Since we have a case of metabolic acidosis we can use Winter's Formula where PCO2=1.5xHCO3+8+/-2=1.5x18+8=32+/-2=30-34
Since our patients PCO2 level was 32mmHg we see that there is an appropriate level of compensation

**Step 5:** Determine the etiology: In this case we have a patient with a Hx of depression who was found in his garage and found to be confused, had vomited, has tachypnea, and has a metabolic acidosis. This begins to paint the picture of intoxication with ethylene glycol. We know that he has a metabolic acidosis from his laboratory data. If this is the case then there must be an anion gap which will confirm our diagnosis short of a blood level of ethylene glycol (which is not always available given instrumentation availability). If we calculate this it turns out to be AG=140-100-18=22 which is well above the upper limit of normal. If we wish to verify this diagnosis even further we can order a urine osmolar gap.

*Sample Case 3:*
A 17 yo girl is brought in to your clinic by her sister because she is concerned about her pronounced weight loss over the last several months and concerning behavior for constant trips to the restroom after meals. This became most concerning today because she made 5 trips to the restroom in the 2 hours after breakfast. On observation she is a shy and thin appearing female in mild distress that is reluctant to discuss her sister's observations. Physical Exam is notable for dental caries in molars. Vitals: Temp 99.8, BP: 95/65, RR=7, Labs: Na138, K3.0, Cl 100, PCO2=50mmHg, HCO3- 34mmol/L, pH=7.55. What is the etiology of her acid base disturbance?

**Step 1:** From the H&P we begin to suspect that this patient has been vomiting. There are several pieces of information from the vignette that point to this diagnosis and let us see as we work through the steps if the data matches our suspicion.

**Step 2:** pH=7.55 is clearly an alkalemia and will now have to elucidate some of the potential causes

**Step 3:** Using the flowchart above we determine that this patient has a metabolic alkalosis because her HCO3- >24mmol/L. Let us check to see is she has the proper level of compensation.

**Step 4:** When using some of the commonly used "rules of thumb" for compensation we expect a 1.0mmHg rise in PCO2 for every 1.0 rise in HCO3-. Thus, for our patient there is an appropriate amount of compensation.

**Step 5:** Determine the etiology: This case appears to be a straightforward case of metabolic alkalosis secondary to vomiting in a patient that most likely is bulimic. She has a history of intractable vomiting evidenced by her alkalosis, hypokalemia, and hypercarbonatemia. She has a proper ventilatory response with hypoventilation and resultant hypercapnea. If we wish to further corroborate our findings we can order a urine chloride test which should show a Cl level less than 15mmol/L. The treatment for a patient such as this will be psychiatric with the possible use of medications.

**Sample Case 4:**

22 y/o college student is brought in to the emergency room at 5am by his friends who stated that he developed drowsiness and has been unresponsive for over an hour. On observation he has miosis, is breathing very slowly, and is not responding to verbal stimuli. His friends tell you that at the party he had been drinking alcohol and "popping some pills". Vitals: Temp 99.0, RR=5, BP=110/85, Labs: ABG pH=7.25, HCO3=28mmol/L, PCO2=60mmHg Chem Na 140,K 4.0,Cl 100.

**Step 1:** From the clinical vignette we can extract some very useful information: He is unconscious, he is breathing very slowly, he has pinpoint pupils and he has an abnormal set of labs.

**Step 2:** pH=7.25 is clearly an acidemia. We must now determine if this is metabolic or respiratory even though it may be apparent from the story.

**Step 3:** To determine if this is metabolic or respiratory in origin we look at the PCO2 and see that it is above 40mmHg and hence it must be a respiratory acidosis We can now check to see his compensation status using some of the formulas above

**Step 4:** To determine the level of compensation we must ask ourselves if this is an acute or chronic case if we suspect that it is respiratory in origin. For an acute respiratory acidosis we determine that the level of compensation is appropriate because we expect a 1.0 rise in HCO3- levels for every 10mmHg rise in PCO2 levels. Our patient meets that appropriate criteria with a pCO2=60mmHg and an HCO3 = 25mmol/L. We can safely say that he is adequately compensated and that there is not a mixed disorder present.

**Step 5:** Determine the etiology: given the clinical history presented and the laboratory findings we can conclude that this patient is most likely suffering from opiate induced hypoventilatory hypercapnea and a resultant respiratory acidosis. We know that opiates act on the resp center in our brain stem and reduce the ventilator drive leading to CO2 buildup and an acidosis. With the administration of Naloxone, an opiate receptor antagonist we can reverse the effects of the opiate.

## Sample Case 5: Respiratory Alkalosis

An avid skier goes on a skiing trip with his family and gets injured on his first day. At the local clinic the physician notices that he is hyperventilating and decides to take an arterial blood gas. On physical exam he is in moderate distress and has tachypnea. Vitals: HR=100, BP=120/90, RR=22 ABG returns pH=7.55, HCO3-=22, PCO2=30mmHg. Chem panel shows Na 140, Cl 100 and K 3.5. What is the etiology of his acid base disturbance?

**Step 1:** From the H&P it is important to note that he is at altitude, is hyperventilating, and that there are relevant abnormalities on his labs

**Step 2:** pH=7.55 and hence he has an alkalemia

**Step 3:** To determine if this insult is metabolic or respiratory in origin just from the labs we need to look at the HCO3- and pCO2. From the low pCO2 we know that this is a respiratory alkalosis. The HCO3 ≤ 24 mmol/L which technically qualified as a metabolic acidosis but we know that this is most likely the proper level of compensation so let us verify this.

**Step 4:** Determine the level of compensation: Since we are suspecting a respiratory alkalosis we can use some of the compensatory formulas listed above. In the acute setting we can expect a 2.0 mmol/L drop in HCO3- levels for every 10mmHg drop in pCO2 and in this case there appears to be proper compensation. If you would like to use a Davenport diagram remember that for a resp alkalosis you move rightward on the diagonal line until you reach a new pCO2 and pH and then as renal compensation kicks in you move down the isobar until you are at a lower HCO3- as the kidney attempts to unload some of that HCO3-.

**Step 5:** Determine the etiology: from the clinical information we have gathered it is apparent that this is a case of altitude induced respiratory alkalosis. When a patient is exposed to low levels of pO2 arterial chemoreceptors kick in and send the patient into ventilator overdrive producing a hypocapnic state. With decreased CO2 levels the equilibrium is pushed to the left and we lose HCO3- and H+. To compensate for the decreased pH the kidney begins its compensatory process by decreasing its reabsorption of HCO3-. Patients can help accelerate this process if they take a carbonic Anhydrase inhibitor such as acetazolamide.

**Sample Case 6:**

28 y/o male is brought into the emergency room by his roommate after he was found lying in his bed unresponsive. There was an open unlabeled bottle of white tablets on his countertop with vomitus covering his clothes and blanket. Physical exam was notable for the patient being unresponsive. Vitals: HR=120 BP=110/85, RR=24 Temp=100.3. ABGs were ordered and they revealed pH=7.40, PCO2=24mmHg HCO3-=18 mmol/L Chem Panel: Na 143 K 3.2 Cl 100. A Chest XRay revealed pulmonary edema. What is the etiology of his acid base disturbance?

**Step 1:** Beginning our assessment with the history and physical we should comment on the fact that this patient was found unresponsive who had vomited. A bottle of unknown medication which he presumably overdosed on was also found. Objective data show physical findings of tachycardia, tachypnea, and some abnormal laboratory results.

**Step 2:** pH= Normal. This is very surprising because this is an acid base tutorial after all. Though we also know that his PCO2 and HCO3- levels are not normal and form these we can deduce a couple of things. First he has a acidosis from his low bicarbonate levels and a alkalosis from his hypocapnea.

**Step 3:** This problem appears to be tricky because it is unlike anything we have encountered before. Here we have 2 processes that are competing for each other; a metabolic acidosis and a respiratory alkalosis. We can deduce that the alkalosis is respiratory in nature, because of his hyperventilation and by argument the acidosis must be metabolic because the resp causes of acidosis or alkalosis can only be unidirectional.

**Step 4:** To determine if there is adequate compensation we must make calculations for the 2 competing problems. For the metabolic acidosis insult we can again use Winters Formula: PCO2=1.5xHCO3+8+/-2=1.5(18)+8=35+/-2=33-37. His actual pCO2 is much lower than this though. We should start to think about a mixed disorder at this point. Because we have a superimposed respiratory alkalosis also we can argue that he is breathing off even more CO2 explaining why the levels are much lower than the compensation would account for. As far as the resp alkalosis we expect the HCO3 to decrease by 2 for every PCO2 drop of 10mmHg. In this case it has dropped past that and for good reason because there is a competing metabolic acidosis stealing away all those valuable HCO3- ions. Lastly, there is a metabolic alkalosis that is occurring because of the vomiting that occurred. PCO2 increases 0.5-1.0 per 1.0 rise of HCO3- per the compensatory formulas. In this case there is clearly no compensation apparent because this is not the primary insult and is important to note that it is a symptom.

**Step 5:** Determine the etiology: Putting all the information together it is apparent that we have a salicylate toxicity issue. From all the information gathered and the arguments made above it should be clear at this point that there are 3 processes occurring. The most important bit of information we derived besides the history that there was inappropriate compensation suggesting a mixed disorder beyond a reasonable doubt (remember some of the caveats listed in the compensation section). We can further corroborate this diagnosis with the useful anion gap calculation AG=25 which is well above the upper limit of normal. Since we have a positive anion gap we can go ahead and calculate the delta delta ratio Δ/Δ=25-12/24-18 =13/6=2.2 which is greater than 2 and thus there is an anion gap acidosis competing with a mild metabolic alkalosis. This is a great example of a mixed case in which we had 3 states competing with each other simultaneously.

# References:

1) WST Thomson, JF Addams, RA Cowan: Clinical Acid Base Balance 1st ed. Great Brittan: Oxford Medical Publications ,1997.

2) Abelow, Benjamin: Understanding Acid-Base. Philadelphia :Lippincott Williams and Wilkins, 1998.

3) Brensilver, Jeff M. and Goldberger, Emanuel: Water, Electrolyte, and Acid-Base Syndromes 8th ed. Philadelphia : FA Davis Company, 1996.

4) Goldberger, Emmanuel: A primer of Water, electrolyte and acid base syndromes, 7th ed. Philadelphia : Lea and Febiger Publishers, 1986.

5) Lowenstein, Jerome: Acid and Basic A Guide to Understanding Acid Base Disorders. New York: Oxford University press, 1993.

6) Collins, Douglas R.: Illustrated Manual of Fluid and Electrolyte Disorders. Philadelphia: Lippincott J.B. 1976.

www.ingramcontent.com/pod-product-compliance
Lightning Source LLC
Chambersburg PA
CBHW051930210526
45473CB00006B/2195